Essential Oils for Depression

I0441519

A proven Guide for Essential Oils and Aromatherapy for Depression And Stress Relief and a better Life

Tonny M Ford, RN, BSN, PHN.

2015

Essential Oils
For Depression

A PROVEN GUIDE FOR ESSENTIAL OILS AND AROMATHERAPY FOR DEPRESSION, STRESS RELIEF AND A BETTER LIFE

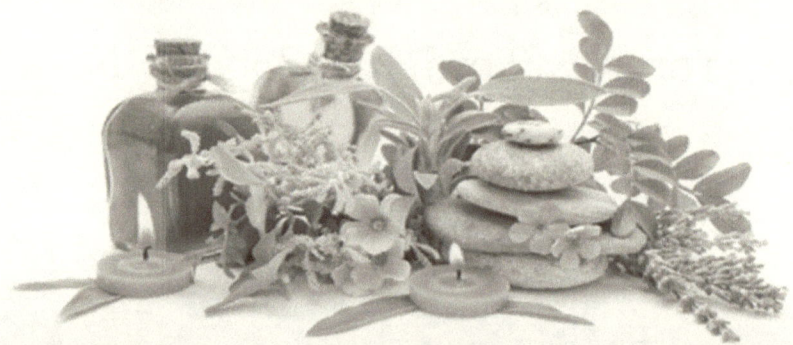

TONNY M FORD, RN, BSN, PHN

essentialoilRN.net

Disclaimer

This book is not intended as a substitute for the medical advice of physicians. The reader should regularly consult a physician in matters relating to his/her health and particularly with respect to any symptoms that may require diagnosis or medical attention.

The information provided in this book is designed to provide helpful information on the subjects discussed. This book is not meant to be used, nor should it be used, to diagnose or treat any medical condition. For diagnosis or treatment of any medical problem, consult your own physician. The publisher and author are not responsible for any specific health or medical needs that may require medical supervision and are not liable for any damages or negative consequences from any treatment, action, application or preparation, to any person reading or following the information in this book. References are provided for informational purposes only and do not constitute endorsement of any websites or other sources. Readers should be aware that the websites listed in this book may change.

Bonus Gift!!

As a way of saying thank you for purchasing our book, we have included a free 140 page exclusive pdf report on **essential oils guide**. We believe that that the value in this report will enrich your life abundantly. As a subscriber, you will the first to get a new free ebooks before anyone else! If you have any questions, please contact us at support@essentialoilrn.net

Click here to download your free bonus ebook

http://www.essentialoilrn.net

Table of Contents

Introduction

I want to thank you and congratulate you for downloading the book, "*Essential Oils for Depression*".

This book contains proven steps and strategies on how to utilize essential oils as remedies for depression and anxiety.

This easy to understand book gives you more information about depression and how aromatherapy using essential oils can help in alleviating the symptoms and eventually helping in the treatment of depression, stress, and anxiety.

This book gives you the knowledge you need about the different kinds of essential oils and the methods that you can use for the treatment.

Readers are also treated to some of the most effective recipes for essential oil blends, diffuser blends, massage oils, and others.

Once you are through with this book, you will be armed with more useful knowledge about essential oils and how it can help cure depression.

Thanks again for downloading this book, I hope you enjoy it!

Chapter 1 Aromatherapy and Depression

Depression

It is normal to be sad sometimes, just it is normal to feel happy. However, sadness or feeling blue should only last for a little while and you will feel happy again after a few days. Not everyone can shake off the "blues" in a matter of days, though, some people may be suffering from depression.

Depression is a common medical condition but it is a serious one. A lot of people who are in a depressive state never seek treatment, either they are not aware that they have the condition or they refuse to seek treatment, insisting that nothing is wrong with them.

There are different kinds of depressive disorders, here are just a few:

- *Major depression* is characterized by severe symptoms that often interfere with one's ability to live "normally" – go to work, or study, sleep, eat, and to basically enjoy life. A person may experience an episode once in their lifetime, but for some people, they experience several episodes.

- *Persistent depressive disorder* is a feeling of sadness and depression that usually lasts for 2 years. Sufferer may experience several episodes but are less severe than major depression. In order to be categorized as persistent depressive disorder, symptoms should manifest for 2 years.

- **Psychotic depression** occurs when one experiences a form of psychosis, like experiencing delusions and hallucinations.
- **Postpartum depression** is more known as "baby blues", wherein a lot of women experience this after giving birth. It happens when women continue to undergo many hormonal and physical changes, including assuming huge responsibility of raising a child.
- **Seasonal affective disorder or SAD** usually occurs during the winter months, where there is less natural light coming from the sun. The feelings of depression usually disappear at the first sight of spring and summer.
- **Bipolar disorder** is often associated with depression, characterized by sudden mood changes, like from extreme highs to extreme lows.

Depression may be caused by several factors – genetic, environmental, biological, and psychological. There are a lot of different ways to treat depression, and one of them is through aromatherapy.

Aromatherapy

Aromatherapy is an ancient Chinese form of medicine that makes use of organic compounds referred to as essential oils to improve a person's mental state, mood, and overall health. The oils are extracts from the different parts of a plant, including its roots, leaves, blossoms and seeds. The extracts can be blended together to produce aromatic scents.

How does aromatherapy works?

No one knows exactly how aromatherapy works, even researchers have no clue. However, a lot of practitioners believe that the chemicals found in these essential oils can trigger the smell receptors found in the nose, which are connected to the areas in the brain that influence your moods and feelings. They can be used as massage oils, added to your baths, room spray, or applied on the skin, among others. Read more on this in the succeeding chapters.

Some examples of essential oils used for depression are:

- Clary sage
- Lavender
- Sandalwood
- Ylang-ylang
- Bergamot
- Basil
- Jasmine
- Rose
- Neroli
- Geranium

Pros and Cons of Aromatherapy

Aromatherapy is an excellent way to de-stress with its relaxing and calming scents. Usage and handling are simple, and they essential oils are expensive.

However, while essential oils are generally safe, some people may experience allergic reactions from them. There are people who can be quite sensitive to strong scents.

There are no clinical studies that can prove to the efficacy of essential oils and aromatherapy in treating depression, especially the severe ones. But many people continue to attest about the calming effects aromatherapy can bring to them. Psychotherapists recommend the use of essential oils in massages and meditation to make them more effective.

Aromatherapy and Depression

Two of the major causes for developing anxiety and depression are situational triggers and hormonal imbalances.

Situational triggers include the following:
- A loved one's death
- Divorce/breakup of a relationship
- Loss of job/opportunity
- Transferring houses or states
- Financial crisis
- Stressful job
- Retirement
- Pressure from loved ones and superiors

Most sufferers wouldn't want to face or do not even realize that they are suffering from depression. For most people, admitting that they have a problem, especially with their health, is a sign of weakness, so they try to stay strong even if they know deep inside that they can no longer handle it. Still there are others who are not aware that they are suffering from depression and anxiety.

It is important that if you feel that you in a lot of stress and pressure, and you have the above conditions, consult a qualified doctor right away. Do not hesitate in going to the doctor. Some people think are embarrassed to be seen going to a psychiatrist because they don't be want to be perceived as one suffering from mental illness, so most people who suffer from even the mildest type of depression end up not getting the proper diagnose and treatment that they need.

The first step is to admit that there is something amiss and the logical second step is to consult a qualified medical practitioner.

There are natural and homeopathic treatments that you can do on your own but it is still important that you consult with a qualified physician or a naturopathic doctor to find out what these treatments are.

In this book, we present aromatherapy and essential oils as treatment for depression; find out more in the succeeding chapters.

Chapter 2 How to Use Essential Oils for Depression

There are a variety of ways to use essential oils to treat depression. This chapter gives you a step-by-step guide on how the methods of preparing essential oils.

Knowing the Type of Essential Oil to Use

Each of the essential oils have been are known to have different effects on people. This is just a rundown of the most popular and commonly used essential oils known to help treat depression and anxiety.

- *Clary sage,* for instance, can be used by insomnia sufferers, in addition to treating depression and anxiety.
- *Rose* targets your entire nervous system.
- *Sandalwood* is known for its sedative properties that can effective alleviate tensions and anxiety.
- *Lavender* is an effective treatment for depression, tension, migraines, headaches insomnia, and hypertension.

You'll find more explanation as you continue to read through the book.

Create an Uplifting Recipe

You can create your own blend of essential oils, depending how you want to use them for depression treatment.

Diffuse

Diffusion is the process of spreading the scent of the essential oil continuously throughout one area. A diffuser is used for this purpose. You can add a few drops of your chosen essential oil to the diffuser. Let it diffuse throughout the day to calm your mind and uplift your spirit. If you want to get a good night's sleep, diffuse it at night in the bedroom.

You may also add a few drops to your pillow so you can inhale the calming scent as you sleep.

Inhalation

This is the easiest way to utilize your favorite scent. Add 1 to 2 drops of your chosen essential oil into your palms, and then rub them together. Cup both of your palms over your nose and take at 5 to 6 deep and slow breaths. This will help change your mood, relieve stress, and make you forget about your anxiety.

You can also use a cotton ball. Just put 2 to 4 drops of essential oil on a cotton ball and place in a zip lock bag so you can take the scent with you as you travel.

You may also bring a small bottle of your favorite essential oil so you can sniff its scent whenever you feel like to.

Air Freshener

You can also create a calming and uplifting air freshener or room spray that is safer and more natural than the commercially-available products in the market today.

You'll need a 4 oz clean spray bottle with fine mist. Make sure that you are not using a recycled spray bottle, especially it contained hair products like hair spray). You can add about 30 to 40 drops of the essential oil of your choice, or you can also use an essential oil blend. (Get more information on this on the next chapters.)

You can simply mix the essential oil with 1.5 fl. Oz. distilled water (you can alternatively use hydrosol) and 1/5 fl. oz. high proof alcohol. You may opt not to add alcohol and just double the amount of distilled water (or hydrosol).

You may use these essential oil blends if you wish:

- 14 drops of bergamot EO
- 4 drops of ylang-ylang EO
- 20 drops of lime EO
- 2 drops of rose EO

Or

- 20 drops of rosemary EO
- 8 drops of grapefruit EO
- 4 drops of peppermint EO
- 2 drops of spearmint EO

Or

- 15 drops of clary sage EO
- 9 drops of lemon EO
- 6 drops of lavender EO

Make sure not to overfill the spray bottle, you need to make sure that you leave a little room for the bottle to shaken. This will also ensure that the content does not float to the very top in between uses.

When you are ready, shake the bottle before every use. Spray light in the room. Avoid spraying directly to your furniture or open beverage containers.

Massage

One of the most common uses of essential oils is during a therapeutic massage. When combined with aromatherapy, a full-body massage helps give you complete relaxation and calmness, helping ease mental and physical stress.

Use 2 oz. carrier oil, add in 10 to 12 drops of your chosen essential oil or essential oil blend and have it used as massage oil when you go out to the spa.

Baths

You can find different kinds of essential oils and salts with oils that you can add to your bath for a relaxing, calming, and therapeutic experience.

Just 5 to 10 drops of your favorite essential oil or essential oil blend added to your bath tub helps ease feelings of depression, anxiety, and stress. If you are prone to allergic reactions, dilute the essential oil in one tablespoon of carrier oil before you add the liquid to the bath tub. Diluting in carrier oil provides moisturizing effect. It also serves as protection to your sensitive skin.

It is not advisable to add in the essential oil to running water because the oil will only evaporate at a faster speed.

Skin and Hair Care Products

There are safe beauty products available in the market today with scented essential oils. These products are great ways to keep the calming scent with you throughout the day.

But you may also consider making your own to ensure that you are using safe product for your hair and skin. You can add in calming, relaxing, or uplifting essential oils that can help reduce the emotional and physical symptoms of depression, stress, and anxiety.

You may purchase unscented products (you may find these in health shops and specialty stores) and add a few drops of your preferred essential oil. There are pre-made products, like shampoos, conditioners, lotions, and bath gels that you can purchase. Just make sure the aroma of the pre-made product will blend well with the essential oil.

Surround Yourself with Your Favorite Scent

There are a variety of ways to do that:

- You can add a few drops of your favorite essential oil to your lotion.
- Take a tissue paper or a cotton ball, put a few drops of your favorite, and place it in the car.
- You can also make your clothes smelling good. Simply add at least 2 drops of your favorite essential oil on a piece of clothing and put it the dryer.

- Smell the aromatic scent while you clean by adding 2 to 3 drops of essential oil on a cotton ball and place in the vacuum cleaner.

Chapter 3 Possible Applications of Essential Oils

Stress, anxiety, depression, and a host of other intense negative emotions deprive us of living the life we want. In this fast paced world, it is hard not to get stressed out. Nurturing these negative emotions is not beneficial to anyone's overall state of healthy.

For those who are looking for an easy and inexpensive way to combat depression, stress, and anxiety, aromatherapy and essential oils are the best choices.

Here are some recommendations on the possible uses of essential oils to alleviate common mental, physical, and emotional issues. See what can work for you.

Anxiety

Inhale a few drops of essential oil that you sprayed on the palms of your hand. Breathe in deeply and slowly for a few minutes until you feel that your mood is changing.

Abuse

The stigma of an abuse, whether physical or verbal is hard to shake off – it brings trauma and fear. This can also lead to depression. You can fight back these emotions. Daily inhalation of your favorite essential oil helps alleviate the anxiety brought about by the abuse. You can also rub your chosen oil on your solar plexus, it is located just above your abdomen.

Relief to Cushing's syndrome

Cushing's syndrome is a collection of signs and symptoms of prolonged exposure to cortisol. Symptoms include high blood pressure, reddish stretch mark, fat lump felt between the shoulders, weakening of the bones and muscles, fragile and sensitive skin, acne breakouts, and abdominal obesity but the arms and the legs are visibly thin.

It also brings about mood changes, severe headaches, and a fatigue.

You can ease the symptoms by massaging 1 to 2 drops of essential oil on the soles of your feet on a daily basis.

Decreased Vitality

It is normal to lose vitality and feel lethargic all the time you are stressed and depressed, brought about my too much pressure at work (or at school). Most of the time you just have to go on because that is what is expected of you and you cannot afford working hard because you want to help in providing for the family.

Refresh and renew your energy by applying 1 to 2 drops of your chosen scent over your chest area where the heart is and on your solar plexus.

Energy

If you are someone who needs to finish a lot of tasks on a daily basis, it is understandable to lose steam towards the afternoon. For sudden perks of energy boost bring with you a small bottle of essential oil and inhale the scent every so often through the day. You can also use a diffuser and place it on your desk to create a calming atmosphere in an otherwise busy work area.

Fear

Fear is a natural feeling by any human being. If you do not feel fear, you won't find the courage to take risks. Whenever you are feeling intimidated, take out your tiny bottle of essential oil and sniff for a couple of minutes until you feel fear is subsiding and being replaced by confidence and calmness.

Grief and Sorrow

Grief and sorrow is inevitable. If you are mourning over a loss of a loved one or a job, do not let it lead to depression, and take action at once. You can begin by applying 1 to 2 drops of essential oils over your heart and your throat. Ylang-ylang is a good choice to be applied over the heart.

Motivation
When you are looking for motivation to finish a given task, gently rub 1 to 2 drops of essential oil over the solar plexus daily or as needed.

Focus
When you are besieged with tons of work, it is hard to concentrate and focus, lest you won't be able to finish your task on time. It is easy to lose focus rather when you think about the tasks at hand, but aromatherapy can address that. Diffuse your choice of essential oil when you are buried deep in your work or homework.

Pessimism
Throughout the day, when you are tired, it is easy to become a pessimist. However, it is important that you keep your emotions in check all the time.
If you need to replace pessimism with optimism, rub a few drops of essential oil at the back of your neck and over your heart. Do so as needed.

When Overwhelmed
It is easy to get overwhelmed when you have a lot of things to do daily. Find calmness and relaxation by spraying a few drops of essential oil into your palms and rub them together. Inhale the scent for a few minutes, inhaling slowly and deeply.

When You Need to Lighten Up
Sometimes you may feel that you are becoming too serious and you have somewhat lost your sense of humor, you can diffuse your favorite essential oil scent all-day-long or you can massage about 2 drops of it over your solar plexus and your heart every day.

Tensed
When there is a project that needs to be done as soon as possible or you have exams coming up, you can become too tensed and worried, which can lead to anxiety and eventually depression. Simply massage about 2 to 3 drops of your choice of essential oils into the areas of your body that feels the tension or massage into the soles of your feet.

Need Uplifting
If you need to feel uplifted, diffuse your favorite essential oil in your room throughout the day or massage the soles of your feet with essential oil.

Worried
Most of the time you might worry about how you can finish a project. Maybe you constantly worry about how you can continue to provide for your family. Worry is a normal feeling but it is not healthy. You can worry about things for a while but you shouldn't dwell on them. To help you ease up a little, place about 1 to 2 drops of essential oil blend on your palms. Bring your palms to your nose and breathe into them slowly and deeply for a few minutes.

There are a lot more things that you can address with aromatherapy. You just need to experiment on the scents of the different essential oils so you can find what's going to work for you.

Chapter 4 The Best Essential Oils for Depression

Aromatherapy makes use of aromatic essences extracted from a variety of plant sources. You can liken essential oils to your hormones – they can control biochemical reactions and send messages between the cells in your body; plus, they protect plants from common bacteria, fungi, and parasites. They are also an important product of the plant source.

Essential oils are strong, actually way too strong to be used directly on your skin. You do not apply the oil directly on your skin. If you are going to use them for massage, you combine with massage oil or a massage cream/lotion. You also do not directly rub oil on your skin when you use it for baths – you will still need to dilute the essential oil on the water.

You have to be aware that there are certain oils that counteract homeopathic remedies. Make sure that you consult with a homeopath before you use them both at the same time.

Aromatherapy can be used to treat mild forms of depression. When used properly, it can help you to sleep better and calm mental fatigue. For more serious forms of depression, you might need a more help that aromatherapy.

Uplifting Essential Oils

Uplifting oils are those that help perk up your mood when you are feeling low. They can "bring you back to your happy place". These include the following:

Bergamot – has a refreshing scent that is uplifting. It also helps you deal with intense feelings of sadness, pain, anxiety, and depression.

Cypress – has a sedating effect that can help relax your mind and body, thus, offering relief from anxiety. It also helps stimulate a happy feeling whenever you are feeling sad or angry. Cypress is used in calming someone who were under a lot of serious shock or trauma.

Lemongrass – is known to repel insects, that it is an important ingredient in insect repellant lotions and sprays. One of the most important medicinal properties of lemongrass is being an effective sedative. When inhaled, it has a soothing effect on the body and the mind. Its fragrant scent helps relieve tension and anxiety. It is also a good cure for insomnia.

Rosemary – helps improve one's mood and it helps boost your memory. It also helps reduce pain and inflammation, and stimulates good blood circulation.

Clary sage – helps in the relief of insomnia, depression, and anxiety.

Soothing Essential Oils
Soothing oils help you relax the mind and body. Their aroma is calming and comforting. They are widely used in perfumes because of their soothing effects.

Some of the most popular soothing essential oils are:

Chamomile – works by relaxing and calming your mind and body. It is often recommended for people who are suffering from depression and anxiety.

Geranium – is a natural sedative that helps lift up your spirit and releases negative thoughts and emotions. It is used to alleviate the symptoms caused by anxiety and depression.

Jasmine – is good for relaxation. Its calming flowery scent has uplifting and antispasmodic properties.

Lavender – is one of the most popular essential oils. It is often referred to as the cure-all essential oil because it can help ease migraine headache symptoms, alleviate fear, nervousness, anxiety, depression, insomnia, and hypertension. It has an overall calming and relaxing effect on your mind and body.

Marjoram – has been used for medicinal purposes for ages. It is known to ease feelings of grief, loneliness, fear, rejection, and anxiety.

Neroli – has been used as sedative, tonic, and anti-depressant. This essential oil is derived from citrus fruit, with a botanical name of *Citrus Aurantium*.

Patchouli – is known for its anti-depressant, tonic, and sedative properties. It has long been known as an effective insect repellant.

Rose – is known for its great flowery fragrance. It has a stimulating effect that can influence the entire nervous system, thus, bringing complete relaxation and calmness. It can give you a sense of well-being.

Sandalwood – has a comforting scent that gives its potent sedative properties, making this essential oil an effective anti-depressant. It helps relieve the symptoms brought about by stress and anxiety.

Ylang-Ylang – is known for its calming and relaxing scent which helps balance female and male energies. The scent of this essential oil is known to restore one's confidence. It brings you back into the right equilibrium. It is also used to treat symptoms of depression and anxiety. It is also popular among insomniacs because its scent can help them sleep better.

You'll get more information about essential oils in other chapters.

Chapter 5 Recipes

It is better to mix your own essential oil blends rather than buying the readily-available ones. You are assured that you are using all-natural ingredients and you can adjust according to the scent you prefer. You can even experiment until you find the one that you prefer.

For Mild Depression
This is an inhalation blend that can help treat mild depression.

Essential oils:
>   4 parts Ylang-Ylang
>   4 parts Clary sage
>   2 parts Basil
>   3 parts Geranium
>   1 part Sandalwood

Mix these essential oils together in a clean amber glass bottle. Make sure you label the bottle, especially if you plan to make different blends; plus you'll know the date of preparation. You can use this 3 to 4 times every day.

Oil Blend for Depression
Essential Oils
>   Clary sage
>   Basil
>   Jasmine
>   German chamomile
>   Rose

Mix these essential oils together. If you are using a bowl of steaming water, use 2 to 3 drops of each kind of oil. If you are using it for your bath, add 5 to 6 drops of each essential oil.

Bergamot-Chamomile Mix

Essential oils:
>4% Bergamot
>6% Chamomile
>4% Jasmine

Take these three on a brown sugar tablet once a day.

Massage Formulation

Massage and aromatherapy are the best combination when it comes to providing complete relaxation. This is beneficial for one who is suffering from mild depression:

Ingredients:
>2 tbsp sweet almond oil (you can also use vegetable oil)
>1 tsp wheat germ oil
>8 drops Ylang-ylang EO
>8 drops Lavender EO
>2 drops Bergamot EO
>2 drops Basil EO
>2 drops Geranium EO

Mix the essential oils in a clean amber glass bottle. Add in sweet almond oil and wheat germ oil. Gently shake. Apply a small amount of the concentrated massage oil on the back of your hands and chest area. You can simply inhale the aroma to ease depression. Do this 2 to 3 times a day.

Aromatherapy Bath to Relieve Depression

This blend will help treat mild depression:

Ingredients:
>¼ cup Honey (you can also use canola, almond, safflower, or soy)
>3 drops Ylang-ylang EO
>3 drops Lavender EO
>2 drops Geranium EO
>2 drops Basil EO
>1 drop Grapefruit EO

Mix together all the essential oils and honey in a glass bowl. Fill your bath tub with warm water. Pour in the essential oils and honey mixture. Mix well with your hands. Soak in this relaxing bath for 20 to 30 minutes.

Basil Blend

Basil essential oil, though not as popular as the others, provides a refreshing scent. It also helps stimulate your senses, especially when you are feeling blue and depressed. Experts also recommend this essential oil to relieve mental exhaustion. It is an effective tool to fight off depression, anxiety, irritability, migraine headaches, and mental fatigue. It also gives you a state of emotional peace and calmness.

Essential oils:

> 7 drops Bergamot EO
> 7 drops Basil EO
> 2 drops Lavender EO
> 1 drop Eucalyptus EO
> 3 drops Peppermint EO

Mix all these together and inhale or use for your bath.

Soothing Blend

Essential oils:

> 3 drops Sandalwood EO
> 1 drop Rose EO
> 1 drop Orange EO

Mix these three together in a clean amber glass bottle. Inhale the essences by applying a few drops on your palms. Take deep slow breaths as you cover your nose with your scented palms.

Soothing Blend Number 2

Essential oils:

> 2 drops Clary sage EO
> 3 drops Bergamot EO

Mix them in an amber glass bottle. Shake gently. Apply 2 to 3 drops to your palms and inhale. You may also add a few drops to a cotton ball and place in the dashboard of your car. You may also add a few drops on your pillow so you can sleep soundly at night.

Ylang-ylang-Lavender Blend

Essential oils:

> 1 drop Ylang-ylang EO

2 drop Lavender EO

3 drops Grapefruit EO

Mix the three together. Gently shake. Use an amber glass bottle. Don't forget to label the bottle.

Soothing Frankincense Blend

Essential oils:

2 drops Frankincense EO

2 drops Jasmine or Neroli EO

1 drop Lemon EO

Mix well in an amber glass bottle and label. Add a few drops on your pillow for the most soothing sleep ever. You may also add a few drops on your palms and inhale the calming scent of this blend.

Methods

You can then select any of these blends, and choose which method you would want to use. Here are the procedures to guide you on what to do:

As Diffuser Blend

- Multiply the blend of your choice by 4 to get a total of 20 drops.
- Add in the essential oil of your choice to an amber-colored glass bottle. Make sure that it is mixed thoroughly by gently rolling the bottle between the palms of your hands.
- Add in the allowed number of drops of the blend you created to your diffuser, this will depend on what the manufacturer's instructions.

As Bath Oil

- Multiply the blend by 3 to get the total of 15 drops of your preferred blend.
- Combine the 15 drops blend to the bath oil recipe (See recipe below.)

Bath Oil Recipe

You can actually directly add-in skin-safe essential oils to your bath, but essential oils and water do not stay mixed and you could risk concentrated essential oil getting into contact with your skin that may cause allergic reactions. It is recommended that you use bath oil.

You'll need:

- 2 fl. oz. carrier oil (jojoba oil)
- 20 drops of lavender essential oil (or 15 drops of your own blend)

Blend them together and store in a clean glass bottle. You can adjust twice or thrice the measurements found in this recipe.

You will use not all the 2 fl. oz. preparation bath oil in just one bath. Once the tub is full with water, add in about ¼ oz. or 8 ml. of the prepared bath oil into your bath water.

Ensure that the bath oil has been dispensed thoroughly in the tub before you soak yourself in. Remember to add the bath oil just before you get into the tub, after the tub is full with bath water. This will prevent the bath oil from evaporating even before you could hop in for a relaxing dip.

As Bath Salts

- You will only multiply the blend by 4 in order to get the 20 drops you need of your chosen blend.
- You may now mix this with the bath salts you prepared. (See recipe below.)

Bath Salts

You'll need the following:

- 3 cups salt (you may use sea salt, Himalayan pink salt, Dead Sea salt, Epsom salt, or you combine any of these salts. Generally, salts have different sizes of grain. When you combine multiple grain sizes, you make the salt more appealing visually. But while chunkier salt types may be more visually appealing, they take longer to dissolve, hence, it might be painful when you step or sit on a few large pieces that didn't fully dissolve.

- 15 to 24 drops of your chosen essential oil (or essential oil blend).
- You may or may not add a tablespoon of any of these oils for added moisture: jojoba or fractionated coconut.

Place salt on a medium-sized mixing bowl. If you chose to add in oil within this recipe, add it to the plain salts and then mix them well. You may then add your chosen essential oils. Don't forget to mix each time you add into the mixture. Transfer the mixture to a salt tube or glass bottle with tight –fitting lid. Take note that if you keep the salts in non-airtight containers, it stands to lose aroma more quickly.
You may add about ½ to 1 cup of the bath salts to running water. Make sure you mix the salts into the water thoroughly. Soak in the tub and enjoy a relaxing bath.

As Massage Oil
- Multiply the blend by 2 in order to get the 10 drops you need of your preferred blend.
- Add this to the massage oil recipe. (See below)

Massage Oil Recipe
You'll need these:
- 1 fl. oz. carrier oil, like sweet almond oil.

- 10 to 12 drops of essential oils. Choose oils that meet the goals you want to achieve with your massage session.

Examples are:
- *Stress blend:* 6 drops of clary sage, 2 drops of lemon, and 3 drops of lavender.
- *Aphrodisiac blend:* 8 drops of sandalwood, and 2 drops of jasmine.
- *Sleep inducing blend:* 10 drops of roman chamomile.
- *Sore muscles blend:* 2 drops of ginger, 2 drops of black pepper, 5 drops of eucalyptus, and 4 drops of peppermint.

Make sure the essential oils are mixed well. Store the mixture in a dark-colored, airtight container. You can have this recipe doubled or tripled, according to what you need.
Apply about ½ to 1 teaspoon of mixture for each massage.

Diffuser Recipes

Included in this chapter are recipes that you can use with your essential oil diffuser. You can create any of the blends of your choice by adding the right amount of essential oils to amber-colored glass bottle. And then you can add in the right number of drops needed from the prepared blend to the diffuser.
It is important that you study and understand first the safety and contraindications for all types of essential oils before you begin handling, processing, and using them. It is ideal to being with the smallest possible amount of blend first, and if you the blend give you the scent and mood that you want, you can double or triple the recipe.

Another important reminder: absolutes and more concentrated essential oils, such as oakmoss, benzoin, verivert, patchouli, and sandalwood, should be handled in nebulizing diffusers. Make sure you read and understand the instructions that come with the diffuser.

These diffuser recipes are developed to create the best smelling fragrances that can effectively change your mood immediately. Keep in mind that they were not formulated to treat a specific disorder or condition in mind. But one thing is for sure, these blends can help greatly with your emotional well-being.

Diffuser Recipe 1

- 5 drops of lime EO
- 3 drops of sweet orange EO
- 1 drop of jasmine EO
- 1 drop of cinnamon EO

Diffuser Recipe 2

- 4 drops of bergamot EO
- 3 drops of sandalwood EO
- 2 drops of grapefruit EO
- 1 drop of jasmine EO

Diffuser Recipe 3

- 12 drops of patchouli EO
- 5 drops of vanilla EO
- 2 drops of linden blossom EO
- 1 drop of neroli EO

Diffuser Recipe 4

- 4 drops of bergamot EO
- 2 drops of lemon EO
- 2 drops of grapefruit EO
- 2 drops of ylang-ylang EO

Diffuser Recipe 5
- 10 drops of lime EO
- 7 drops of bergamot EO
- 2 drops of ylang-ylang EO
- 1 drop of rose EO

Diffuser Recipe 6
- 5 drops of spruce EO
- 3 drops of cedar EO
- 2 drops of lavender EO

Diffuser Recipe 7
- 5 drops of lavender EO
- 4 drops of rosewood EO
- 1 drop of ylang-ylang EO

Diffuser Recipe 8
- 5 drops of rosemary EO
- 3 drops of lavender EO
- 1 drop of roman chamomile EO
- 1 drop of peppermint EO

Diffuser Recipe 9
- 11 drops of lemon EO
- 6 drops of bergamot EO
- 3 drops of spearmint EO

Diffuser Recipe 10
- 5 drops of bergamot EO
- 4 drops of lavender EO
- 1 drop of cypress EO

Diffuser Recipe 11

- 9 drops of sweet orange EO
- 5 drops of lavender EO
- 5 drops of spearmint EO

Diffuser Recipe 12
- 5 drops of sandalwood EO
- 2 drops of lemon EO
- 2 drops of scotch pine EO
- 1 drop of rose EO

Diffuser Recipe 13
- 6 drops of sweet orange EO
- 3 drops of patchouli EO
- 1 drop of jasmine EO

Diffuser Recipe 14
- 7 drops of sweet orange EO
- 2 drops of vanilla EO
- 1 drop of ylang-ylang EO

Diffuser Recipe 15
- 4 drops of clary safe EO
- 4 drops of ylang-ylang EO
- 2 drops of bergamot EO

Diffuser Recipe 16
- 9 drops of sandalwood EO
- 1 drop of neroli EO

Diffuser Recipe 17
- 6 drops of juniper EO
- 3 drops of sweet orange EO
- 1 drop cinnamon EO

Chapter 6 Essential Oils to Uplift Your Mood

Depression and anxiety, though common, are quite complicated. Emotional disorders are difficult to discuss. It is hard for the sufferer because most of them are not comfortable on revealing their condition.

Most of the time, a few therapy sessions would help treat the disorders. Some people, though, always look for the alternative and natural remedies. In the previous chapters, it has been discussed how essential oils and aromatherapy can help you if you are suffering from depression.

The following list includes three of the most potent essential oils that help cure depression.

Bergamot – The Mood Booster

Bergamot or *Citrus aurantium* or *bergamia*, is a strong essential oil that has been known to effectively help treat depression. The citrus family is known for their uplifting effects, and bergamot is recognized as the most powerful. There are many anecdotal and historical narratives about its potency, particularly as an antidepressant. There are recent scientific studies conducted among 58 patients that showed interesting results. The respondents were given hand massages daily for a week, using a blend of 1.5% dilution with almond oil. The essential oil blend contains the following: bergamot, lavender, and frankincense, in equal ratios. Scientists conclude that all of the patients who received the aromatherapy hand massage exhibited lesser pain and decreased depression symptoms. However, they didn't conduct other tests with the use of other essential oil samples. Hence, the only conclusion that can be derived from this study is that aromatherapy massage using the essential oil blend is proven to be more effective in easing the pain and managing the symptoms for depression, than simple massage alone.

There is also a study conducted to find proof that lavender can treat anxiety and depression. Focusing on the psychological stress signals, researchers selected people who are known to be exposed to a lot of stress at work. The participants were administered bergamot. Results showed that a short 10-minuteinhalation of the essential oil weekly is enough to significantly reduce high blood person and bring a person's heart to normal. It also was evident that those who had high levels of depression and anxiety benefited to the tests.

You can try this *anti-stress blend*:
Essential Oils:
>   5 drops Lavender EO
>   3 drops Ylang-ylang EO
>   2 drops Bergamot EO

Mix these three essential oils in an amber glass bottle. Put about 3 drops to your bath and soak in warm water for 20 to 30 minutes. You can also use it as to soak either foot or your hands daily, best done before you hit the sack. If you don't have a tub, you can add a few drops into your liquid bath soap and douse it as you shower every day.

Clary Sage – Keeping You Calm and Clear

The term *clary* was derived from the Latin word *sclarea*, derived from the word *clarus*, which means "clear". Aromatherapy practitioners would like to believe that the name, clary sage or *Salvia sclarea* essential oil actually means "clearing away the dark clouds caused by bad mood". Clary sage has long been used to help uplift one's spirit. It gives you feelings of euphoria when you use it regularly.

This one-of-a-kind essential oil can be diffused in your room just before you go to sleep to give you the most relaxing and rejuvenating sleep ever. You may also add a few drops to your bath and soak in the warm water with clary sage between 20 to 30 minutes and you are surely to come out relaxed and blissful.

Are there scientific basis to its claims? There have been several studies conducted to verify if clary sage can effectively turn your bad mood into a good one. Researchers have discovered that clary sage has antidepressant properties, thus, it can be used treat anxiety disorders and depression.

Try this relaxing bath blend if you must:
Essential oils:
>   3 drops Clary sage EO
>   2 drops Ylang-ylang EO

Combine these two essential oils. Mix it well. Add to your bath, make sure the tub is full with warm water before you mix in to bath blend – you don't want to have it evaporating before you can even soak yourself in. Immerse in that relaxing bath for 30 minutes. Feel the calming and cleaning effect the essential oils give to your warm bath and get out of it refreshed and ready to take on new challenges.

Lavender: The Ultimate Symbol of Peace and Tranquility

Lavender is probably the most popular essential oil used for relaxation. Its scientific name is *Lavandula angustifolia*. Aside from possessing a heavenly scent, it is considered to be a versatile flower (or herb) and essential oil. It can be used for a lot of things, including support for people suffering from insomnia, promote healthy and positive mood, relaxation, and even pest control, among other things.

The main concern here now is, is it any good to help treat depression? Experts and aromatherapy practitioners say that it is. A study shows that the condition of patients tested who are suffering from mild to moderate depression exhibited marked improvement after being administered 60 drops of lavender tincture daily.

Another study further gives proof to its potency as anti-depressant. That same study showed that aromatherapy using lavender essential oil effectively reduced serum cortisol levels, which help triggers your body's negative response to stress. Researchers strongly concluded that lavender essential oil have powerful relaxation properties and beneficial in coronary circulation.

Further studies are being conducted to find more proof to the theory and initial findings that lavender can be an equally effective substitute for drugs used to treat anxiety because lavender is not addictive and 100% natural. In fact, there is also a research wherein scientists investigated the use of lavender essential oil for patients diagnosed with Generalized Anxiety Disorder or GAD.

An approved medication called Silexan is an oral lavender oil capsule preparation. Patients with GAD were asked to take Silexan in lieu of other medications for 6 weeks, and these patients manifested relief from anxiety symptoms. It is also important to take note that Silexan is safe and non-addictive. It has no known sedative effects compared with other drugs. However, you need to be aware that *lavender L. angustifolia* is not the same as *lavandin Lavandula intermedia*. Lavender has potent relaxing properties while lavandin has stimulating effects. When you are using lavender essential oil for the purpose of relaxation purposes, it is important to remember to check the name of the product and/or raw essential oil you will be getting, it has to be *Lavandula angustifolia*.

Chapter 7 More Essential Oils and Their Benefits and Uses

Aromatherapy is a versatile holistic treatment. The use of all-natural essential oils is a good addition to therapeutic massage, bath massages, diffusers, and all the other techniques.

In this chapter, you will learn more uses for some of the widely used essential oils that can be used as natural anxiety and depression relief.

Valerian Root
Valerian is a perennial flower that is found in most parts of Asia and Europe. The United States have started growing valerian plants of late. Scientific name is *Valeriana officialis*. While it has been used because of its delectable fragrance for more than 500 years, its medicinal benefits have just been found out for centuries.

Valerian root is known for a variety of health benefits, such as:

- Reduce heart palpitations and irregular heartbeat.
- Improve the quality of sleep.
- Protect the skin from irritants.
- Lower high blood pressure.
- Ease gastrointestinal problems.
- Reduce nervous breakdowns.
- Stimulate cognitive skills.
- Lessen menstrual cramps.
- Ease depression and anxiety symptoms.

It has been referred to as a "heal-all" plant. Valerian essential oil has terpenes, alkaloids, and flavonoles.

Valerian root essential oil can be mixed with pine, patchouli, and pine. In general, there are no known negative side effects from using valerian root essential oil; however, the presence of several powerful but volatile components, you don't need much to experience any side effect. Excessive consumption of this essential oil may lead to dizziness, mild depression, stomachaches, cramps, and skin rashes. But reports of side effects are uncommon.

Tangerine Essential Oil

Tangerine is a member of the citrus family. Tangerine fruit is almost similar to the mandarin oranges, only tangerine has a deeper color and lacking in pips. It is scientifically known as *Citrus reticulata*. It grows abundantly in China, and from there, this beneficial fruit has spread all over the world. It has been used by the Chinese for its medicinal properties for decades.

Benefits include:

- Works as antiseptic. Tangerine essential oil contains components that kill *Staphylococcus aureus* bacteria, which causes sepsis. The oil can be applied topically to open wounds or taken orally.
- Tangerine essential oil contains components that help stimulate the production of new cells, cell division, and the recycling of cellular materials in the body.
- Provides relief from body pain and spasms.
- Helps soothe inflammation in the body's organ systems.
- Boosts your body's immune system and metabolism.
- Purifies the blood and flushes away harmful toxins.
- Keeps your skin moisturized.
  Tangerine essential oil blends well with bergamot, clary sage, clove, lavender, frankincense, nutmeg, neroli, and cinnamon, to aid in the treatment of depression and anxiety.

Basil Essential Oil

You probably know basil as used in cooking, but its leaves and seeds are known to have medicinal benefits. It is abundant in Central Asia, India, Southeast Asia, and Europe. The oil is used extensively for cooking purposes in the Mediterranean and is also a major ingredient in pasta recipes, particularly pesto.

Basil has been used in the ancient times in India mainly as ayuvedic medicine.

Benefits include:

- Relief from symptoms of depression and anxiety.
- Helps improve your skin tone and serves as protection from acne breakouts.
- Helps in the treatment of flatulence, constipation, and indigestion.
- Helps improve the circulatory system.
- Relief from pain.
- Used to treat insect bites and bee stings.
- Helps prevent nausea and vomiting due to motion sickness.
- Treats mental fatigue.
- Eases migraine headaches.

Basil essential oil blends well with other essential oils that improve moods and treat depression, like geranium, clary sage, bergamot, neroli, and lavender.

Eucalyptus Essential Oil

Eucalyptus essential oil is extracted from the fresh leaves of the evergreen eucalyptus tree. Scientific name is *Eucalyptus globules,* and is also referred to as blue gum tree, stringy bark tree, or fever tree, depending on where in the world it is grown. Eucalyptus originated from Australia, but has spread throughout India, South Africa, and Europe.

Its medicinal properties have been recognized, thus, it has become available as primary ingredients to over-the-counter drugs and other medications, like rubs, liniments, inhalers, mouthwashes, and rash creams.

Heath benefits of eucalyptus are:

- Because of its antiseptic properties, eucalyptus essential oil is used in spas and saunas. Its vapor has soothing and calming benefits.
- Helps ease muscle tension.
- Eucalyptus provides relief from mental fatigue. Most people use this essential oil due to its refreshing and cooling effect when applied.
- It helps rejuvenate your tired and sluggish mind and body, thus, it has been considered as an effective treatment for depression and anxiety.
- Helps treat skin infections.
- Boosts your body's immune system.
- Helps relieve influenza symptoms.

Its use in aromatherapy is now growing in popularity. Eucalyptus essential oil blends well with lavender, frankincense, and cedar wood.

A word of caution though, excessive amounts can be toxic. It can interfere with other homeopathic treatments and cause allergic reactions. It is important that you consult with your doctor first if you are prone to allergies or you are undergoing other treatments.

Coriander Essential Oil

Coriander is more popularly known as a kind of spice for different cuisines, but it is also widely used because of its medicinal benefits.

Coriander essential oil is extracted from its seeds through steam distillation. Scientific name is *Coriandrum sativum*. The essential oil is composed of compounds like Cymene, Linalool, Terpinol, Dipentene, Borneol, and Terpinolene. Heath benefits are:

- Relief from stress, depression, and anxiety.
- Relieves spasms and cramps.
- Helps stimulate hormone and enzyme productions and functions.

- Eliminates excess gas.
- A good detoxifier.
- Helps purify blood.
- Improves your appetite.
- Helps in weight loss.
- Inhibits fungal infections.
- Increases sexual libido.

Coriander essential oil blends well with cinnamon, neroli, orange, lemon, grapefruit, ginger, and bergamot.

When taken in excess, coriander essential oil may cause you lose control over your senses for a time, it is like entering a trance or becoming "spell bound". It is a powerful agent that impacts the mind so you have to take extra care in its use.

Lime Essential Oil

Scientific name is *Citrus aurantifolia,* lime essential oil is consists of compounds: Alpha and Beta Pinene, Mycrene, Cineole, Borneol, Neral, Acetate, and Terpinolene.
Health benefits include:

- Provides relief from stress and depression.
- Helps reduce muscle and joint pains.
- Helps restore energy levels.
- Helps in the fight of viral infections.
- Promotes blood coagulation.
- Helps delay the aging process.
- Helps treat food poisoning and typhoid.

Lime essential oil can be mixed with lavender, ylang-ylang, neroli, and clary sage essential oils.

Jasmine Essential Oil

Jasmine is a popular flower with a strong but sweet and romantic scent. It is in bloom only at night. Jasmine primarily grows in the Middle Eastern region and in India. Jasmine is known in two scientific names, *Jasminum grandiflora* or Royal Jasmine and *Jasminum officinale* or Common jasmine.

Oil is extracted from the flowers, mainly consists of benzoic acid, benzyl acetate, benzaldehyde, benzyl alcohol, benzyl benzonate, indole, phytol, and more.

More than its sweet smell, jasmine has incredible health benefits:

- Its aroma is uplifting, so it helps fight depression and anxiety. Its sweet smell makes you feel happy and opens up your romantic and even poetic feelings. The smell of jasmine essential oil in the room stimulates the production of hormones in the body, particularly serotonin, the "happy hormone".
- Jasmine essential oil is also used as disinfectant and antiseptic. It contains benzoic acid, benzyl benzoate, and benzaldehyde, which are known to have powerful germicidal, fungicidal, antiviral, and bactericidal properties.
- It helps get you a restful sleep.
- You may not know it but jasmine essential oil has aphrodisiac properties. It sets people in the mood for love and enhances sexual desires.
- It restores moisture to dry or dehydrated skin. It is used to treat dermatitis and eczema.
- It is an effective treatment for cough.
- It helps reduce labor pains in women. However, pregnant women should avoid this essential oil before the birthing process.

Jasmine essential oil is highly sedating and relaxing, thus, you have to avoid using heavy doses. If you are allergic to the flower, you should not use the essential oil.

It best blends with these essential oils: rose, orange, grapefruit, lime, lemon, sandalwood, and bergamot.

Frankincense Essential Oil

Frankincense or Olibanum trees (*Boswellia carteri*), is associated with religious rights, specifically in the Christian tradition. However, frankincense essential oil has a lot of medicinal benefits:

- It is a potent sedative; hence it helps induce feelings of relaxation, mental peace, and spirituality. It helps ease stress, anxiety, and depression. It also induces insight, making you more introspective. Its aroma promotes deep breathing.
- It helps reduce high blood pressure.
- It helps delay the aging process.
- Frankincense oil is an effective antiseptic.
- Helps improve the digestive process.
- Boosts your body's immune system.
- Helps alleviate menstrual syndrome.
- Helps facilitate healing of wounds.
  While the use of frankincense essential oil is generally safe, it is not be used by pregnant women.
  It can best be combined with orange, lemon, lime, lavender, pine, sandalwood, myrrh, and bergamot essential oils.

Bay Leaves Essential Oil
There are several types of plans whose leaves are called "bay leaves", however, the "real bay leave" is the one that is now scientifically as *Laurus nobilis*. The other "bay leaves" are similar in aroma and appearance but they don't contain the same nutrients. This laurel plant grows in abundance in the Mediterranean region. It is an evergreen shrub. Laurel bay leaves have been used for cooking and medicinal purposes for thousands of years.
Here are some of its medicinal benefits:
- Laurel bay leaves, similar to thyme and basil, contain linalool which is known to lower the level of stress hormones through aromatherapy. Bay leaves essential oil helps calm you down and keeps you relaxed even in the most stressful situations.
- Bay leaves have a unique mixture of organic compounds and antioxidants, like phytonutrients, parthenolide, and catechins, which give protection to the body from harmful free radicals. These free radicals cause your healthy cells to mutate into cancer cells, thus, it is safe to say that bay leaves essential oil can help prevent cancer.

- It helps reduce inflammation from joint pains due to arthritis.
- It also helps lower bad cholesterol levels.
- Helps enhance the digestive process and nutrient absorption.
- Helps maintain healthy hair follicles.

Neroli Essential Oil

Neroli is an essential oil from another citrus fruit.
Did you know that Eau-de-Cologne is traditionally made from neroli essential oil? The neroli name has always been related to perfume.
Aside from this, there are medicinal benefits to using neroli essential oil:

- Neroli essential oil helps you cope with depression and anxiety. Its aroma and sweet essence can help uplift your mood and give you a feeling of happiness.
- It works as sedative.
- It is a proven aphrodisiac. It helps cure frigidity, erectile dysfunctions, and impotence. It can bring back your desire for sex.
- It is an excellent disinfectant. It helps treat infections in the urinary tract, kidneys, prostate, and colon when taken orally.
- Neroli essential oil boosts your immune system.
- It promotes proper blood circulation and boosts your body's metabolism.
- It helps provides relief from spasms.
- It helps stimulate cell generation and helps maintain the health of existing ones.
- It is used in anti-mark applications which help erase spots and scars.
- It helps keep skin moisturized and protected from infections. Neroli essential oil can be blended with all kinds of citrus oils; as well as with sandalwood, rosemary, ylang-ylang, geranium, jasmine, and lavender essential oils.

Patchouli Essential Oil

Patchouli essential oil has long been known as an excellent insect repellant. It is only in the last few years that its medicinal properties have been discovered and listed below are just some of them:

- Patchouli essential oil is huge when it comes to treating symptoms of stress, anxiety, and depression.
- It helps soothe inflammations due to fever, and it provides relief from fever as well.
- It is also an excellent antiseptic, protecting wounds from ulcers and infections.
- Patchouli essential oil can be used an aphrodisiac.
- It also promotes cell generation and helps in the production of red blood cells, thus booting your energy levels.
- It is known to treat skin diseases, like eczema, sores, dermatitis, and psoriasis.
  It mixes well with lavender, myrrh, geranium, clary sage, and bergamot essential oils.

Conclusion

Thank you again for downloading this book!

I hope this book was able to help you to finally find relief for depression and anxiety. You'll find that this book is easy to follow and understand. The ideas here are basic, hence, you can easily apply everything that you have learned from reading this book.

The next step is to begin preparing and applying what you have learned. It would also be a good idea if you can educate your family and friends about the benefits of using aromatherapy and essential oils as treatment for depression.

Finally, if you enjoyed this book, then I'd like to ask you for a favor, would you be kind enough to leave a review for this book on Amazon? It'd be greatly appreciated!

Click here to leave a review for this book on Amazon!

Thank you and good luck!